# The Story Book Drink Book

# The Story Book Drink Book

## A Selection of "Dewey Drinks"

This book is all about dear friends of mine.

## Dewey Henry

Strategic Book Publishing and Rights Co.

Strategic Book Publishing & Rights Co., LLC
USA | Singapore
www.sbpra.net

For information about special discounts for bulk purchases, please contact Strategic Book Publishing and Rights Co. Special Sales, at bookorder@ sbpra.net.

ISBN:978-1-950860-82-1

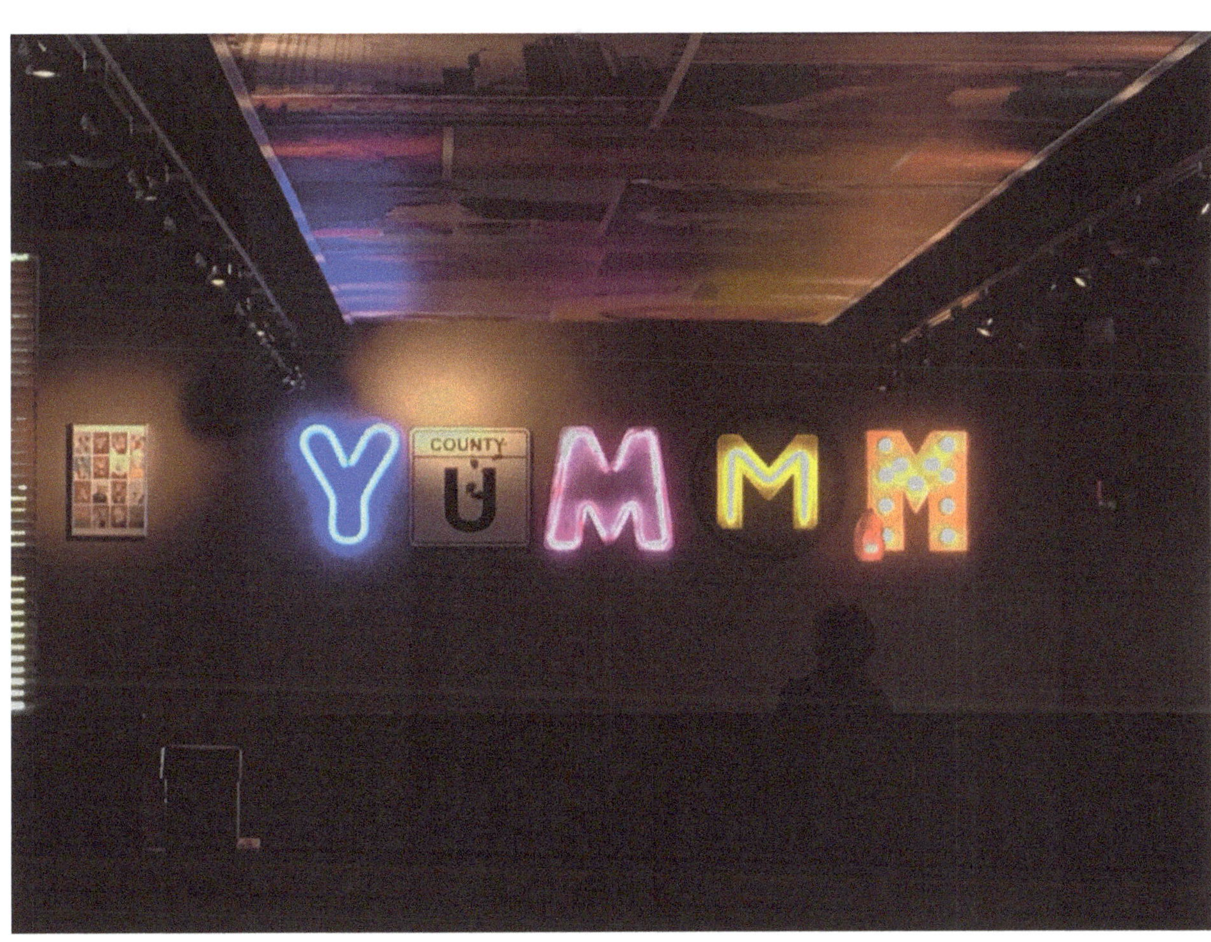

COUNTY

# Preface

I often think of myself as a proud person. Sometimes your pride gets in the way, but most of the time *it is the way!*

Well, I am proud to say that I am a boozer. Yes, that's right, I said *boozer*. Not a drunk or an alcoholic, but a boozer. Do you enjoy a beverage of choice? I know I do, that's for sure.

This is a series of stories of how I came up with the names of drinks that are based on friends. Some came about when I was … well, boozing. Some of them came to life when I was cooking. We like to have a cocktail while cooking. Cooking and booze have been going together for a long time, sometimes in the meal and sometimes in the cook. Ha! Either way, it's always better.

The bartending profession has been in my life for too many years. It's been very good to me and has let me experience many things in life, so I decided to put together this drink book.

Oh, by the way, I am Dewey Henry. Truly my pleasure to meet you. I guess you actually get to meet me. I hope the pleasure is the same for you as it is for me. I really don't know what we just said, but you are going to find out how I talk as you read. Many have said that the way I talk is known as Deweyism!

# Just a Few Deweyisms

| | |
|---|---|
| Boozer: | Someone who is known to have a drink or several |
| Boozing: | Well, someone who is drinking |
| Loopy: | A person who is drinking maybe a bit too much |
| Zippity Do Da: | A shot |
| I Believe I Could Have More: | What I say when I want another |
| Hit Me: | Well, what I say when I want another |
| Just a Splash: | What I say when my wine glass needs refilling |
| I Don't Want to Work Tomorrow: | My favorite wine! (Get it?) |
| Zinger: | A really good shot |
| Barley Pop: | Just a beer |
| Blue Can: | My favorite type of beer |

**Deweyisms with a twist of "Bra"**

| | |
|---|---|
| Bra: | A word that might be used in any way shape or form |
| Brah: | The way my buddy spells it—he's a big dumb animal |
| Braski: | A person snow skiing |
| Bro: | The past tense |
| Brie: | Cheese, you silly people |
| Broheme: | My great friend V |
| Li'l Bra: | An inexperienced bra |
| Brotho: | Someone you are close to but not a relative |
| Braloni: | Any lunch meat that you are eating |
| Bralishish: | Something that is tasty |
| Pinot Noir Bra: | My favorite wine |
| Ya Bra: | A response for everything |
| Brada: | The designer line from bra |
| Nada Brada: | To answer no |
| Bra-zil: | A country in South America |

Okay I think it's time I explained "bra" to everyone. Okay, my great friend uses this term all the time. It truly works for any word. Always used to be funny or witty. Either way, it has become a part of this guy's persona. The bra!

# Southern Style Redneck Martini

- ► 6 oz of good vodka

- ► 1 oz hot pickled okra juice

- ► 1 hot pickled okra

- ► splash of hot sauce

- ► martini glass

- ► shaker and strainer

First and most important is to chill your glass. Put ice in the glass and let it chill for a few minutes. Throw the ice out. Put some ice in a shaker and add the vodka and okra juice. Shake until the ice is bruised. Add a splash of hot sauce to the glass. Strain the liquid into the glass and garnish with the hot okra. Choose any type of okra and your favorite hot sauce, okay, Bo!

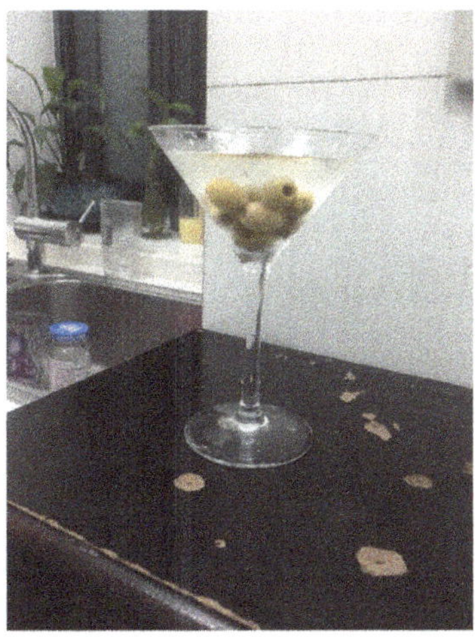

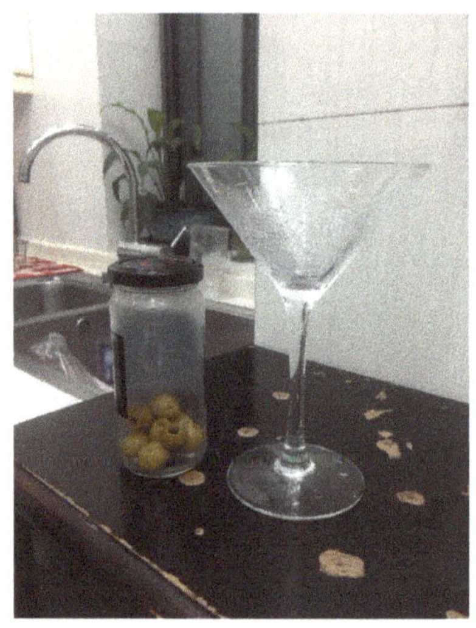

This summer we were fortunate to be able to visit with our friends again. Each year is always different but always better. When we leave, there are stories to be told. Fun events!

Well, here is one of the many that happened this year. I walked into the house of people who were dieting. That subject included the intake of alcohol. My man, AL, was having the hardest time with the diet I think but handling it, as he does. I could only imagine what his thoughts had been for the past ten days. He spoke to me about how he was going to finish the diet, and then have himself a drink that he called a redneck martini. At first, I didn't give it a thought or ask questions.

As the days grew closer to the time for the drink, so did my interest. What could it be? Now, I am not sure that he is a redneck or even knows how to describe one, but my friend sure is trying to be one or definitely has the makings of a redneck in a good way. I think there are all types in all parts of the world.

So the day has finally come, and I get to try a new drink. I have to say I liked it, and it fits his personality too. So, if you are feeling a little red and want a martini, give this beverage a try. I think you might like it too!

# The Root Beer Fistler

- ► 4 oz of vodka

- ► 1/2 oz of Galliano or Florentino (just a splash if you will)

- ► 6 oz of coke

- ► a small beer mug

- ► shaker and strainer

Fill the shaker glass with ice and add all the ingredients.

Shake for a few moments and strain into a shot glass. Use a small version of a beer mug if you can. The key to this beverage is to get that silver frost on it, which happens when you shake and serve it immediately.

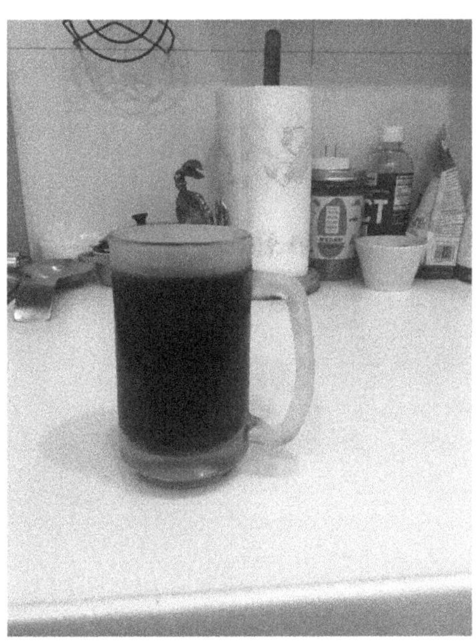

There seem to be things that I can remember, even if they happened yesterday. Then there are things I can't remember at all. Do we really have a selective memory? Or is just that we don't want to remember those things at all? I really don't have the answers to those questions, but I do remember the day I came up with this shot. Well, who really knows if I came up with it because, as I always say, there is no such thing as an original idea. I do keep trying, and I think you should too.

I have to ask, who likes root beer? I think we all do, so I believe if we had it in shot form, we would all drink it.

I was working at this bar, and people were always asking me to come up with a new shot for them. So I was thinking of a frosty root beer with alcohol in it. It was an immediate hit. There was nothing to making many at a time. The phrase was, "a round of root beers for the bar." Who would have known I was a pioneer? Okay, my man, Fistler, came up with the recipe.

# Adam Murphy

- 4 oz of vodka of choice
- 8 oz of half sweet and non-sweet tea
- 16 oz or pint glass
- wedge of a lemon

It's very important to fill the glass to the rim with ice, which is called "packed with ice." You must put the vodka in first, because of its density to the tea. That's all bull, because it doesn't matter at all. However, what really matters is the amount of sweet and non-sweet tea. It totally has to be half and half. Mix well and drink well.

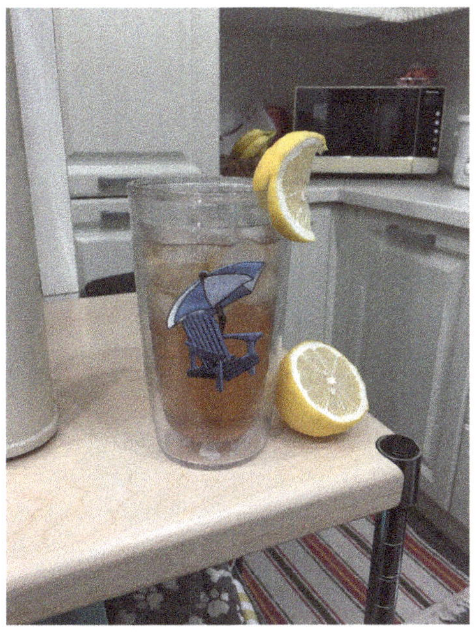

Often I meet people who are just simply cool. I would hope people would want to be cool to me as well. I met a couple of dudes the other day that were just that—cool. I'm under the impression that these guys have known each other for a while; however, I don't know if they were childhood friends. I do know that they will be lifelong friends, and I hope I will be as well. I really don't care if that's sappy or not. So, I made up this drink for two guys who are *pallies* but are also different from each other, kinda like the tea in the drink.

You see, in this crazy world we live in, it's all right to be a li'l bit different from others. If this wasn't true, than I would have no friends! I hope this drink becomes a namesake hit. I believe we should all order one at every bar we go to so we can see if it catches on. The newest sensation in the nation!

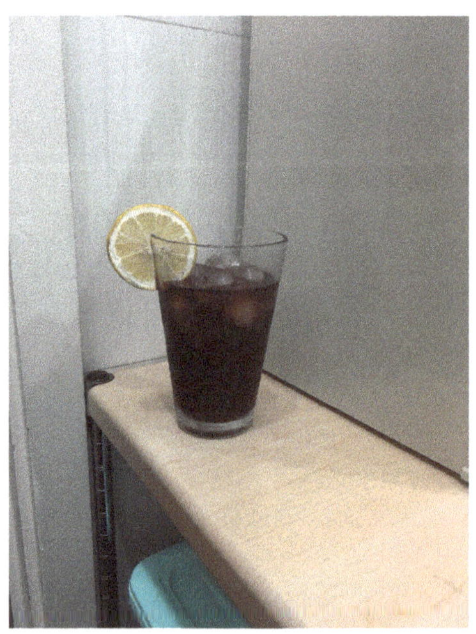

# Yummy Rummy

- ► 4 oz light rum
- ► 4 oz of dark rum
- ► 2 oz orange juice
- ► 2 oz of cranberry juice
- ► 2 oz of pineapple juice
- ► splash of coconut water

I love the tropical feel of this drink. It's as simple as just mixing all of the ingredients together in a big glass. To garnish this drink, you get to choose which fruit you like the best on that particular day. If you want flavored rum, you may use that as well. Either way, it's still yummy.

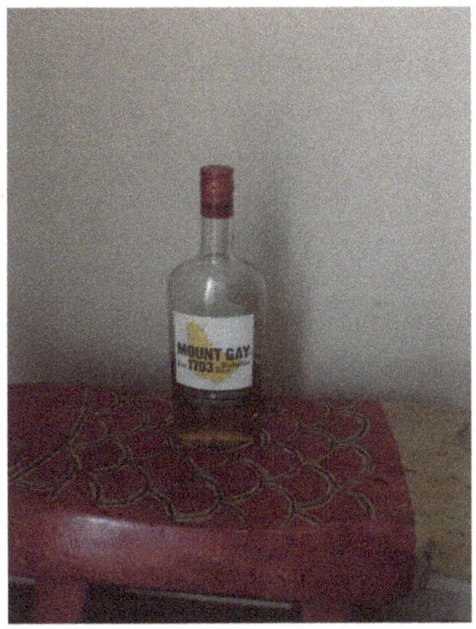

I'm always asking my wife what she would like to eat or drink and seem to get the same answer. It is as follows: "I don't know what I want. I just know what I *don't* want." Wow, that drives me insane, but she's worth it. She does say it just has to be something yummy. Well, duh, I ask you, am I going to make something that's awful? No, I tell you. That's how a beverage like this is available, because there is nobody in the world that can mess it up. It can be made any way you want for all to enjoy.

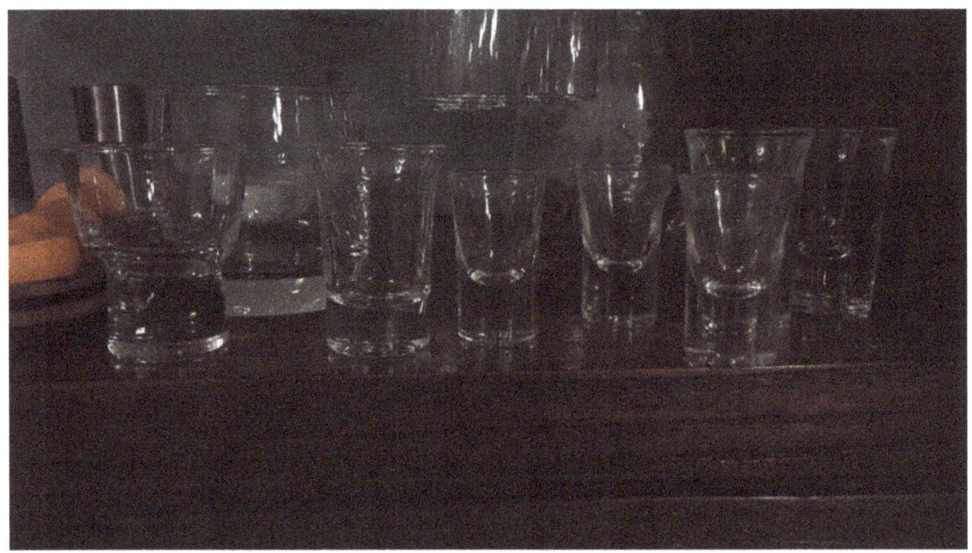

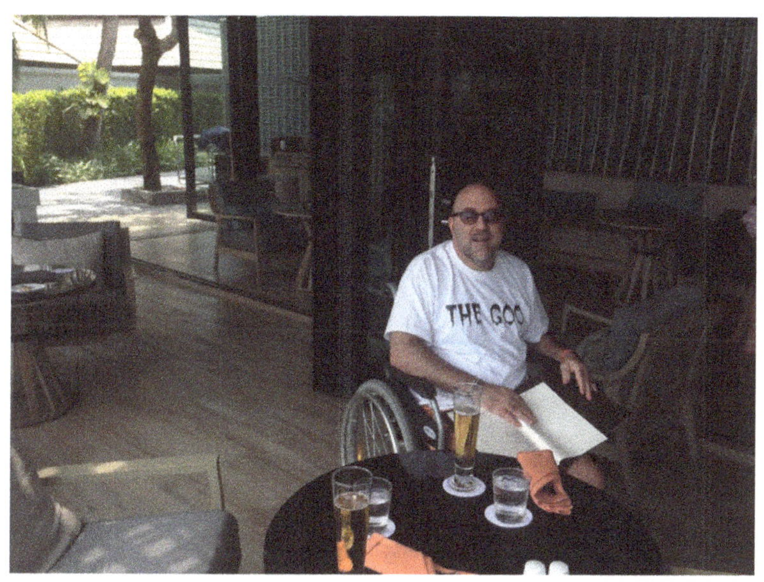

# # 1 Sun

- a really good respido tequila

- a good agave nectar

- a better than average orange juice

- a splash of Grand Marnier

- a Tervis tumbler

There is always a key to a great drink. It's this key that makes the difference between a good drink and a great drink. Try to figure out what the key is to this one. All the stuff that goes into making it includes love. Ya, brotho.

A few years back I married the best girl in the world. The one for me, you know. Not only am I happy with her, but I also got the best mother-in-law. You don't hear people say how great their mother-in-law is or speak highly of her. I'm here to tell you to do so. I know it's a package deal when you get married. I guess I got lucky. Well, I will take it.

Oh, back to the story: So my mother-in-law calls me the "number one son"'cause I married into the family first. She's not the oldest daughter, and I'm not the first one to be introduced as a boyfriend, but I am the first to marry into the family. Therefore, my brother-in-law is known as number two! Ha! Get it? It's funny but, truth be told, *he* is the best son-in-law. I want to make it clear that she calls me number one.

When we all get together, it's a hoot when we talk about this subject. More important, I got to join an awesome family and create a drink that is inspired by the best mother-in-law in the history of mothers-in-law and moms. Ironically, she doesn't even drink!

# A Murphy Adam

- ► (not a black and tan)
- ► half Murphy's stout
- ► half Sam Adams
- ► cold pint glass

It's as simple as it sounds: half of each beer in a cold glass

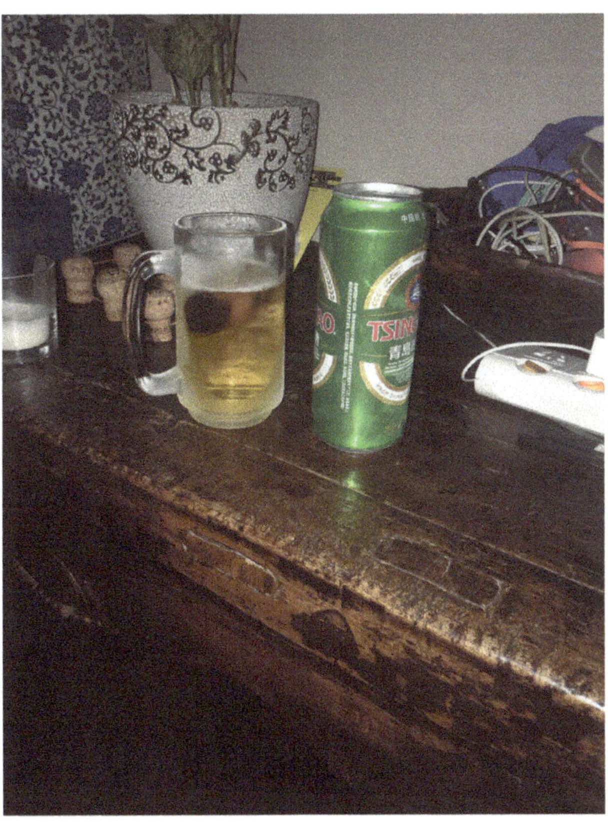

I mostly feel real blessed in life. Especially so when I meet new people who are cool. I was fortunate enough to have this happen to me last week. I met a couple of dudes who I believe have been friends for a while. I hope I get to be friends with them for the rest of my days. These guys couldn't be any more different in style, which I like, because they get on so well. I was thinking that what this crazy world needs the most these days is for all of us to get along. This is why I created this simple blend of beers. It's simply just two unlike things getting along for our refreshment. I believe that's all it takes to enjoy this simple thing called life.

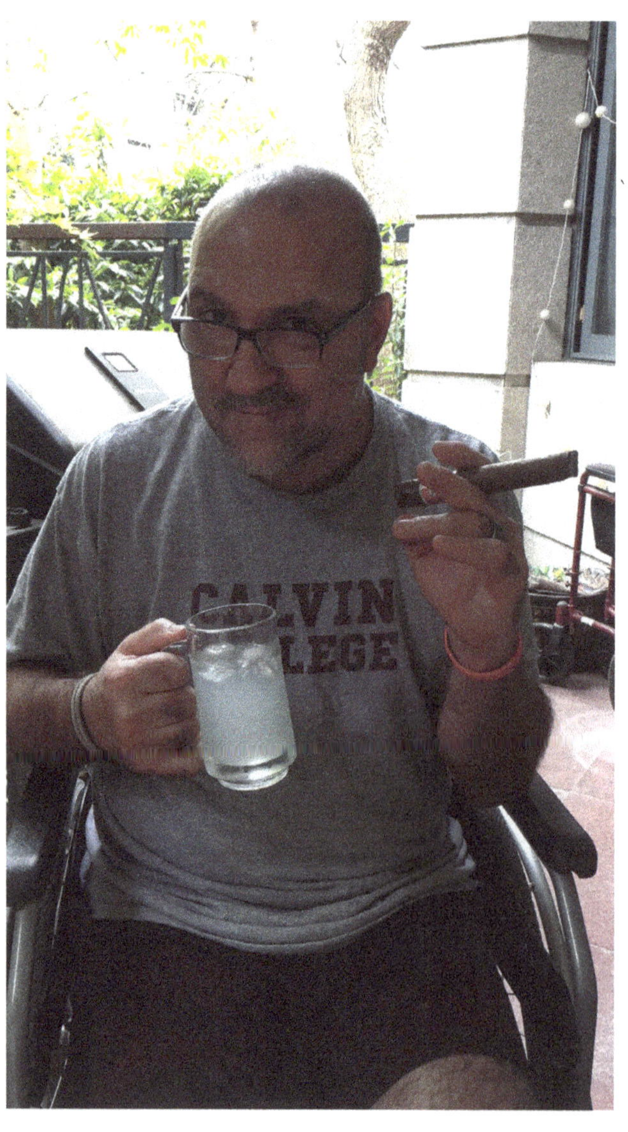

# Old Dewey Henry with a Murphy Adam

The P J
(no, not pajamas or peanut butter and jelly, but my pal Phil Jones)

- ► 7 oz scotch
- ► 7 oz milk

Not only is the name simple, but so are the ingredients. However, if you like your drinks stronger, by all means.

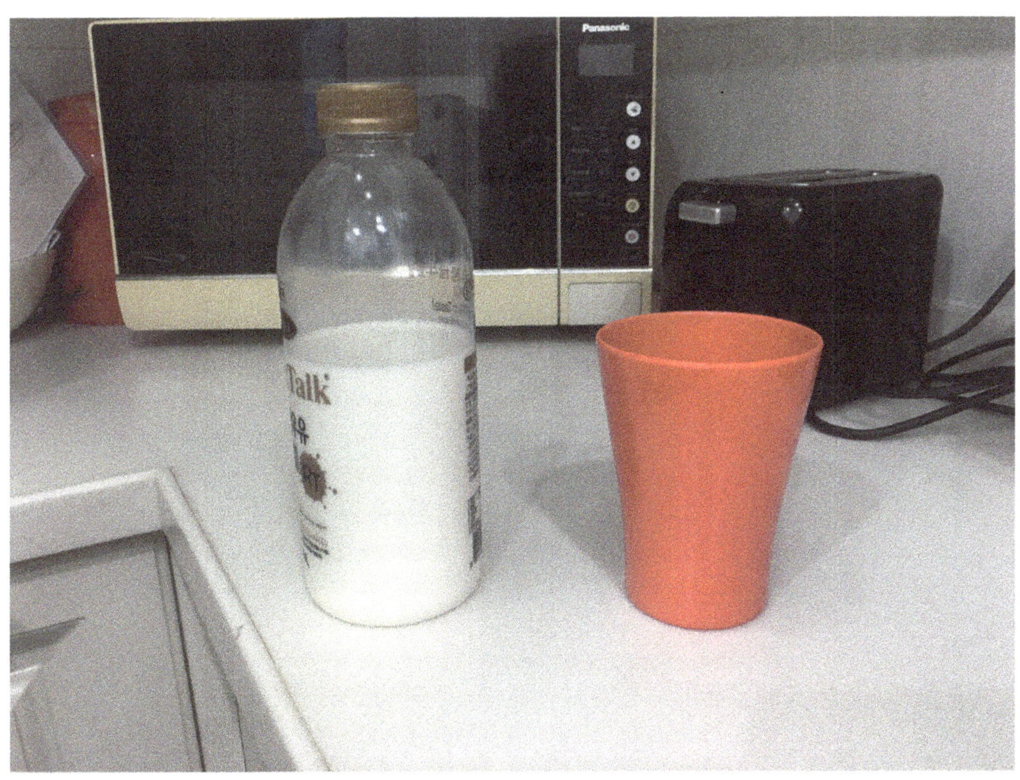

I have a great friend who happens to be a great golfer. One day we were playing a round, and it was very hot out. I suggested we go for a beverage afterwards. Off to the beach bar we go. When we got there, I saw him talking to the barman, also a friend, in a secret, quite soft voice. This was striking me as a li'l bit funny, so I asked the twenty-fifth letter of the alphabet: Why? Get it, Y? Okay, enough of the jokes (there be will more later). His answer was that he wasn't feeling so great and wanted something to make him feel better. To me it was not a problem. What I didn't know was that he had ordered a scotch and milk. However, it had to be in a plastic cup, that way no one would know what he was drinking. It's a big mistake trying to keep something like that from us. It wasn't that long before everyone in the bar knew what he was drinking. Not much longer after that, we all were having one too. I guess we all had upset stomachs.

Here's to you, my friend.

# QIAJ

(Qatar in a Jar)

- a lot of Old Monk rum
- a splash of coke
- a Mason jar
- a li'l bit of ice

This is a strong drink served over ice and it is awesome. It's as simple as putting all of the ingredients in the Mason jar.

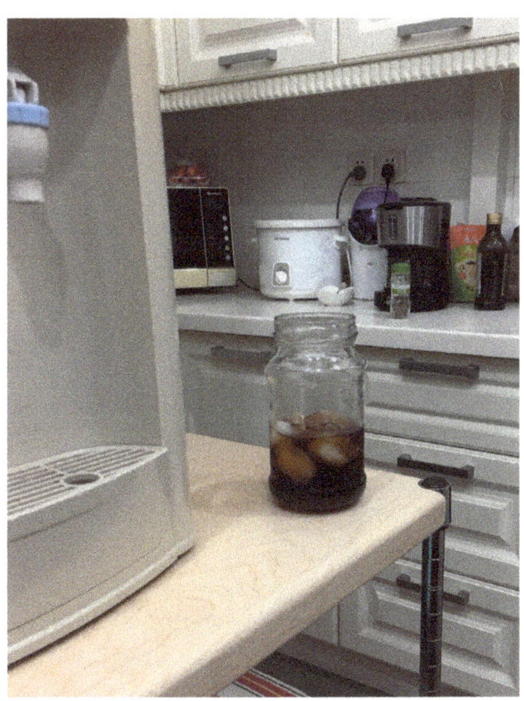

I have a friend who has many nicknames. One he is not called often is Old Monk. It has nothing to do with being old, which he is not, or with being a monk, which he is not. It's just the booze he chooses to drink. It sort of fits him—the name that is. We believe he chose this booze because it is so cheap. Some say he is too, but I don't … well, not to his face anyhow. He gets a little loopy when he drinks Old Monk; however, this is when the best stories happen. Some I might tell and some I will just keep to myself. Either way, my pal is quite entertaining and is very loyal.

Oh, by the way, this guy is my doppelganger. People often get us mixed up. I'm just a little better looking than he is; however, I probably have a bit of an Old Monk in me. The fun we had with people was awesome. The double takes that happened made me laugh as did my old buddy simply known as Old Monk.

To you, pal! "Who the %&@# could be knocking at the door now?"

# Gin SLIM

- ► 4 oz gin
- ► 8 oz strawberry lemonade
- ► pint glass with ice
- ► a li'l bit of mint

You know this is a difficult one. Just mix and serve.

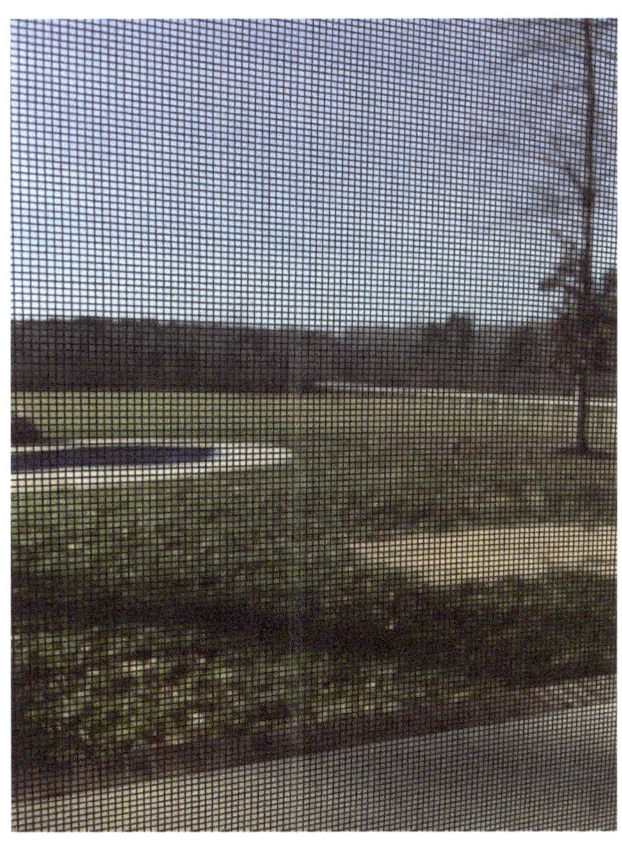

Anyone who knows me understands that I'll use acronyms. Well this is one. The gin is easy; however, the other I will tell you: Strawberry Lemonade, Ice, and Mint equals SLIM. My great friend told me how she liked gin. I like vodka, so I didn't have any gin recipes. Usually vodka drinkers don't drink gin and gin drinkers don't drink vodka. So I thought I would switch the two. This didn't work. I felt like I was short changing all.

Marlene deserves more, because she never would short any one, ever. That's just the type of person she happens to be. I have known many people in my life, and she is top draw. Oh, she is kind of slim and tall, which is, in fact, what you want in a drink. If you are a fan of gin with sweetness, then this is for you, just like my friend, who is one of the sweetest people in world. I truly believe that a person of that nature makes all the difference. The difference between good and great is her. It's all okay. My wife and her husband are very close friends too.

# Keep Your Chin Up

- ► 2 oz rum
- ► 2 oz vodka
- ► 2 oz gin
- ► 2 oz triple sec
- ► splash of sour mix
- ► splash of grenadine

This beverage is similar to another beverage; however, it tastes like lemonade, pink-looking lemonade. Put it in a bigger glass than you imagine, 'cause it will catch up to ya.

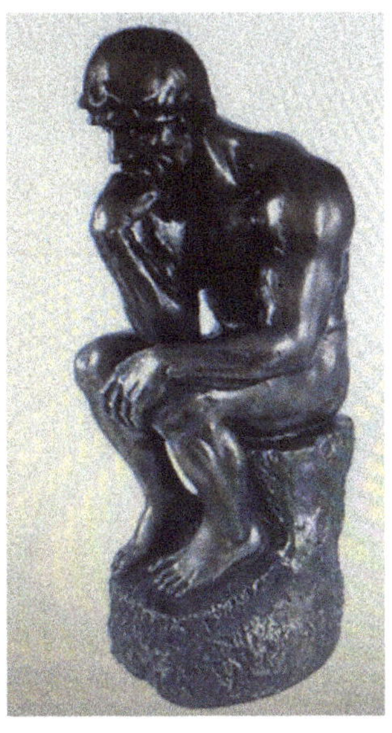

My friend seemed to be hungover when I talked to him over the phone about golfing one morning. In fact, it seemed more than just a hangover. Well, it was. Apparently, he kind of lost his footing while walking the dog. His dog is awesome, however I think the drink might have something to do with it.

So the story goes that, as he was walking the dog, the leash got all twisted up in his legs. My friend's legs, not the dog's legs. He lost his balance and fell right into the mailbox, chin first. Now, why he was checking his mail I have no idea. Once again the *mail*, not to see if the dog was *male*. I am funny! Okay, what's not funny is the fact that he did hurt himself pretty bad. My friend, not the dog, for all you doggie lovers. He did get stitches on that chin, so, the moral of the story is that when drinking, always, and I mean always, no matter what the beverage of choice is to you, you must …

Keep Your Chin Up

# The Wolterman

- ► 2 oz vodka
- ► 2 oz gin
- ► 2 oz soda water
- ► 2 oz tonic water
- ► lemon slice
- ► lime slice

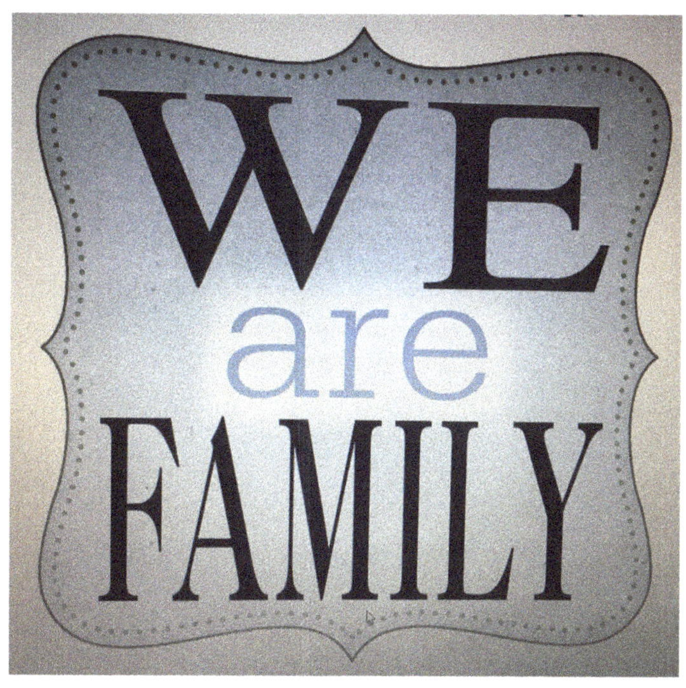

The day this drink was discovered was a very exciting day. There were a bunch of us going out, which added to the excitement. My buddy, Steve, was really geared up for the evening. He kept saying, "What am I going to drink tonight? Gin and tonic or vodka soda? Or maybe something else?"

I wouldn't say he was driving me nuts, 'cause that's the way he is. One of the greatest men I know, so we have to take people for who they are and see the good in them. He did become very successful as he grew older, which I always believed he would. I'm proud to say he is my friend.

Now, I do have to tell you that this drink already has a name. It is called a Charlie Brown. Steve reminds me a bit of that good ole Charlie Brown. There is only one Charlie Brown, and there is only one Wolterman. Like I said, I'm so glad he is my dear friend.

I want to say hello to all of his girls: Maggie, Claire, Ellen, and Nora—The Wolterman Girls!

# 3-5-7

- ► 3 parts lime juice

- ► 5 parts Cointreau

- ► 7 parts tequila

- ► splash of sour mix

- ► splash of orange juice

Now, it's important to understand that when I say "parts," it simply means measurements of all parts. It's up to you if you want to use ounces, liters, bottles, or gallons. If you have a big container, I *bet* you will use the biggest barrel you got! So, *call* all your friends and *raise* your glasses to a toast to three, five, and seven.

99408553463784940004
09814284645555244442
12345678900987654321

For some time, I thought I was the coolest guy on the planet. Until I met my friend, Dan. He's just good enough at all things. Things that matter, you see. For instance, a great Christian, a family man (father and a husband), and teacher of humanities in our middle school molding the futures—that's what I call children at that level of education and age, 'cause that's what they represent. This guy is doing just that for humanity.

Now, you might say he's perfect, but hold on. On poker night he taught us this game he called three five seven, which, I believe, he made up. That's okay, but he also made up the rules as we went along.

I was skeptical at first, but then it was such fun! We had such a great time that I named this drink after him and his game. Okay, mostly after him, because it does match his style: sophisticated and thought worthy. I see this quality in very few people, so it's with great pride that I can call him a great guy and a dear friend. Just don't play poker with him. Ha ha!

# Mandarin Merrill Margarita

("Triple M")

- half bottle of tequila
- 1/4 bottle of Gran Gala
- 8 oz of lemon-infused simple syrup
- juice of 3 limes
- juice of 3 mandarin oranges
- splash of brandy

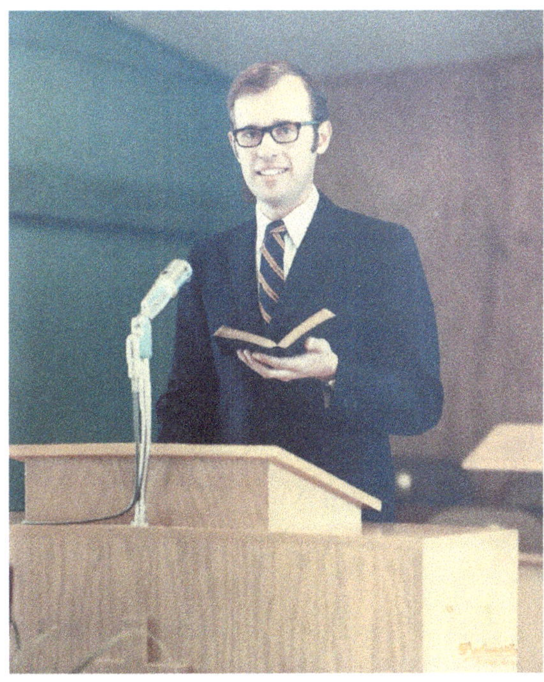

Never would have believed that I would use the term "BFF." However, it applies to this man. I can't really remember when we met or that first conversation, but I know it had to be great, because through the years our chats have been remarkable.

Yes, I know *remarkable* is a strong word. You have to meet my buddy to understand. He's a preacher by trade, which is one of the reasons I learn from him. More knowledge of any and all things learned through education and experience. He's lived an incredible life that he shares with humanity. He is not your ordinary preacher. He's as comfortable up front in the church on Sundays as having a cigar and drink with me. Heck, with anyone. We joke, we laugh, we pray, we talk sports, and discuss and fix world problems without judgement. It's so easy and simple to be around Reverend Timothy. Our beautiful wives work together and are very similar, as we are. Therefore, he and I are usually in trouble. It's worth it, BFF!

# Kahlua Egg Crème

(aka Krumland)

- ► 4 oz Kahlua
- ► 6 oz milk
- ► 4 oz soda water
- ► 2 tbsp of chocolate sauce
- ► pint glass

First off, the glass is essential. Why? Because I said so! Mix all of the ingredients together in order. Why? I believe you know why. Ha. No ice is required, okay?

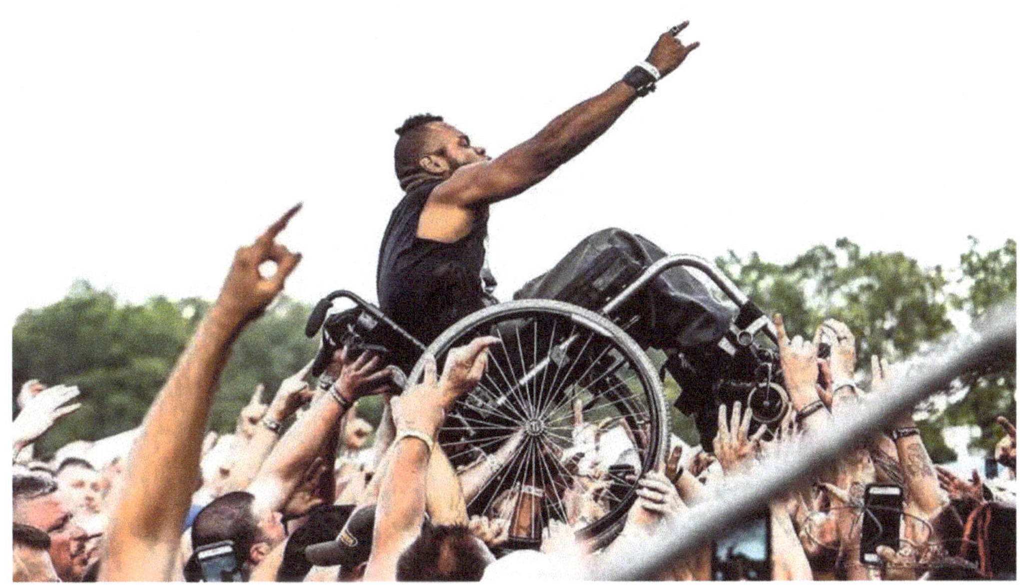

This drink was invented in Brooklyn in the fifties without alcohol. Why? We'll never know. So, I changed it for my good friend, Andrew, because he is always reinventing ways to handle situations. Brilliant, I tell you. Judging from outward appearances alone, you would never think so. But it's what is inside and how you handle yourself that counts.

Now, we all know who Steve Jobs and Bill Gates are. Their outward appearance would never show their brilliance. However, we would be intimidated by them. My man, Andrew, is just as brilliant at things, but somehow never makes anyone feel intimidated. Like I said, brilliant because it's all about the students he helps. I think the egg crème drink is exactly kind of intimidating to try because, who wants a beverage with eggs or crème? Or both? So, I think we have to listen to people as oppose to judging. Andrew does this with brilliance, without a doubt.

Try this drink and, while you're enjoying it, think a lot of personas.

# A Buck

- ► 2 oz Southern Comfort
- ► 2 oz vanilla vodka
- ► 2 oz coke
- ► tall glass with ice

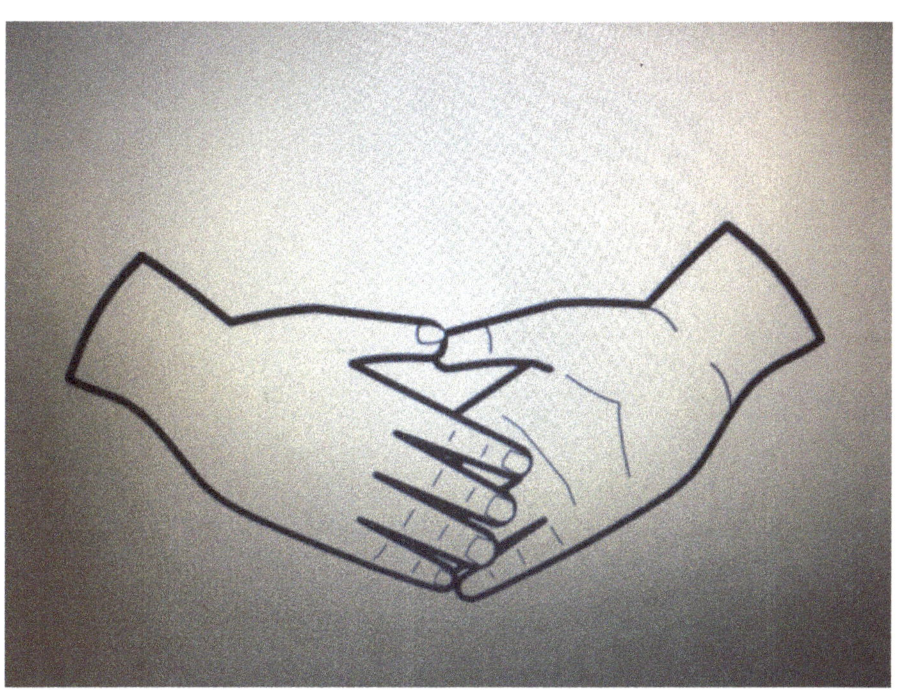

My brother-in-law's brother, Buck, is my bra without a doubt. I met him in the Caribbean at his brother's wedding to my wife's sister. A destination wedding is so awesome. People are always in the best moods. I have to say that when I met him, it was hard to believe that he could ever be in a bad mood. His wife is the same way. It was a short trip and we just got to know each other. However, I do remember a thing he said to me. We wanted to do a shot, so we asked the bartender what we should have. The bartender said, "How about vanilla vodka?" and I said, "How about Southern Comfort?" Buck said to me, "You know what? You're pretty cool." Now I have to say that the shot was terrible. For it was not chilled. My and Buck's friendship is chilled. For many years now. Corrie, his wife, is awesome as well. Their three kids are great. I want to see everyone say to the bartender, "Give me a Buck."

I hope you will make a friend just as I did, a friend who is now family.

# Van Jeano

- ► half of a glass of Prosecco
- ► splash of cranberry juice
- ► splash of orange juice
- ► served in a champagne glass

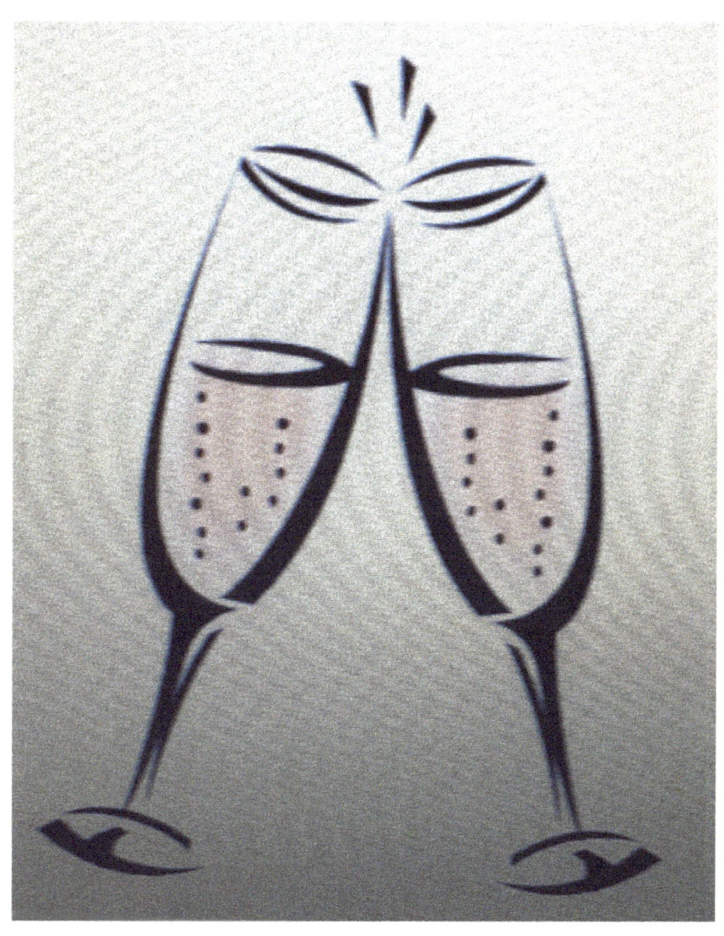

This particular drink is perfect at brunch but can be enjoyed at any time, just like I enjoy the two people it's named after: a grandmother and her first born grandchild. The woman joined our family in the middle of the seventh decade in the twentieth century—that's 1975 for you folks playing at home—and was affectionately known to us simply as Mehall, her maiden name. Yes, she married my brother by choice. Why, I'll never understand. But she is awesome. Some thirty years later, Van was born. A welcome addition. Van is now six years old I think and quite the character!

A story here about Van. He and I were eating cereal one morning while watching cartoons. He finished his and proceeded to place his bowl on the coffee table. I said, "Hey, that doesn't go there." As he leaned over me with a wink and smile, he said, "Jeano will get it." Like I said, he's a character just like the rest of us. Jeano is the only sane one. God bless her!

# Monkey in a Tree

tall, tall, tall, tall, tall glass filled with ice.

- ➤ 2 oz vodka
- ➤ 2 oz gin
- ➤ 2 oz rum
- ➤ 2 oz tequila
- ➤ 2 oz sour mix
- ➤ 2 oz cranberry
- ➤ 2 oz orange juice

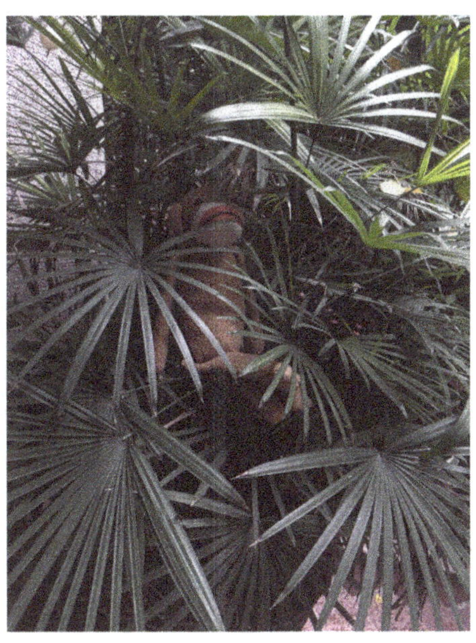

Garth, Garth, Garth, Garth, Garth, and just one more Garth. I can hang with my Garth all day and not be bored. This guy married my niece Annie. You know when it's right. Well, this is right. They are like peas and carrots or like the monkey in a tree. I don't have to explain peas and carrots to you, but I should explain the monkey in the tree.

Annie is the tree. Grounded, rooted. Tall and provides shade for others. She can branch out if she needs a challenge. Her foliage, no matter what time of year, is always beautiful.

Garth is the monkey. Ha! He's not really, but he tries to be, making people laugh with his wit. Truth be told, he is what I call solid, not a monkey. He's so knowledgeable, loyal, great at his job, a provider, a family-first man, a calm person, and, like I said, witty and humorous. He and Annie are great assets to this world. Even my brother trusts Garth.

By the way, they are parents to Van, so you see their characteristics.

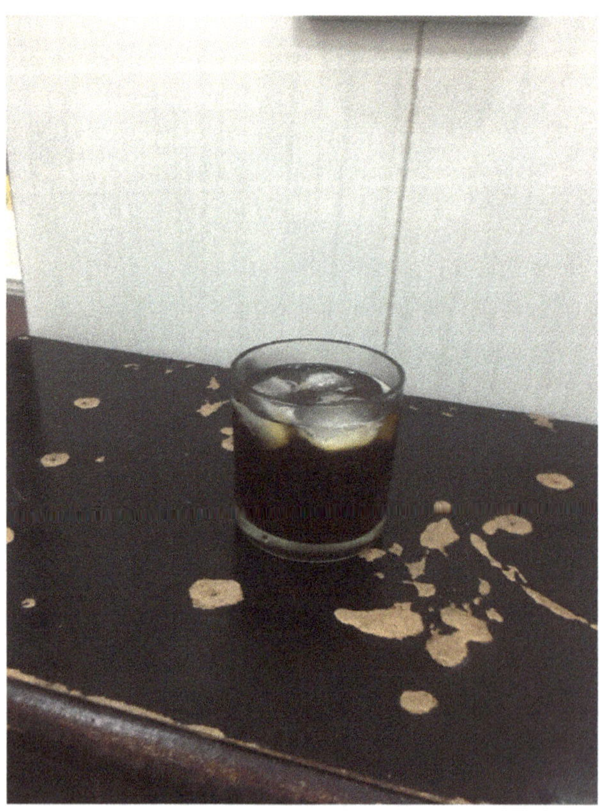

# MacMuffin

► Jack and coke

► any size glass, and as many as you want

► Green Label or even diet, it's your call

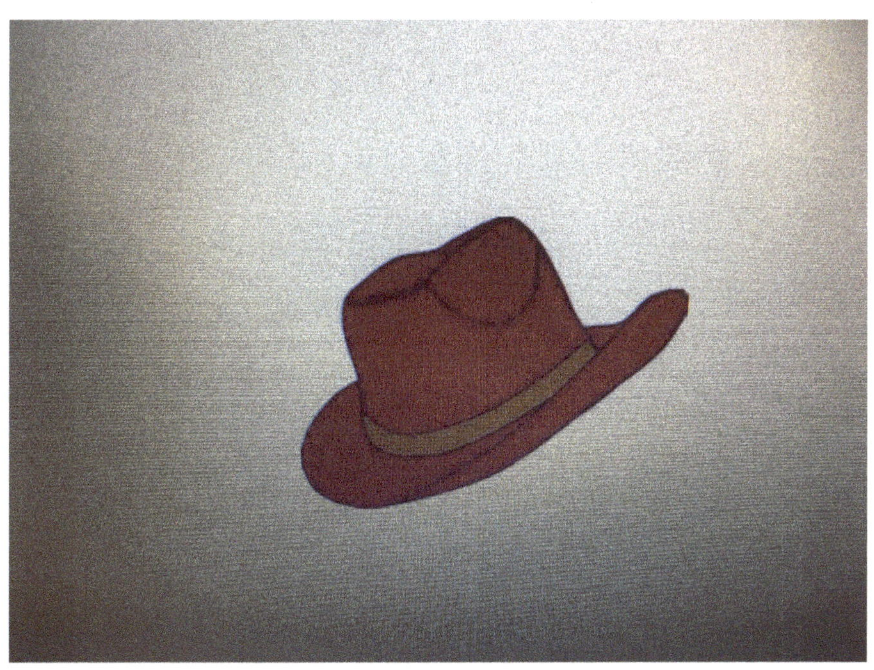

I don't call this guy MacMuffin; my brother does. It's just his way of saying he likes you. His name is Kyle, and he is a good man. Kyle married my niece Callie, and I approve. So does my wife, and that's worth its weight in gold. I happened to be around when they started dating, so of course he was reserved and a li'l bit quiet, which my family is not, including myself. Me, quiet? That's funny. So, we're all hanging out, and I hear Kyle whisper to Callie, "Is your uncle drunk?" She said, "No, he is not. He's always like that. Always!" We had a good laugh at that and have been laughing ever since. This guy is so sincere that it never surprises me when he does something kind, because it's who he is exactly. Exactly! You know, my brother really approves of Kyle for his baby girl. That is also worth its weight in gold.

Kyle, love you, bra. I know you will always take care of family. Okay gang, here's the test: Are you man enough, like my bra, to order a MacMuffin from a bartender? Say Kyle sent you, okay?

# Wheow

- ➤ 4 oz vodka
- ➤ 4 oz orange juice
- ➤ 4 oz soda water
- ➤ pint glass filled with ice

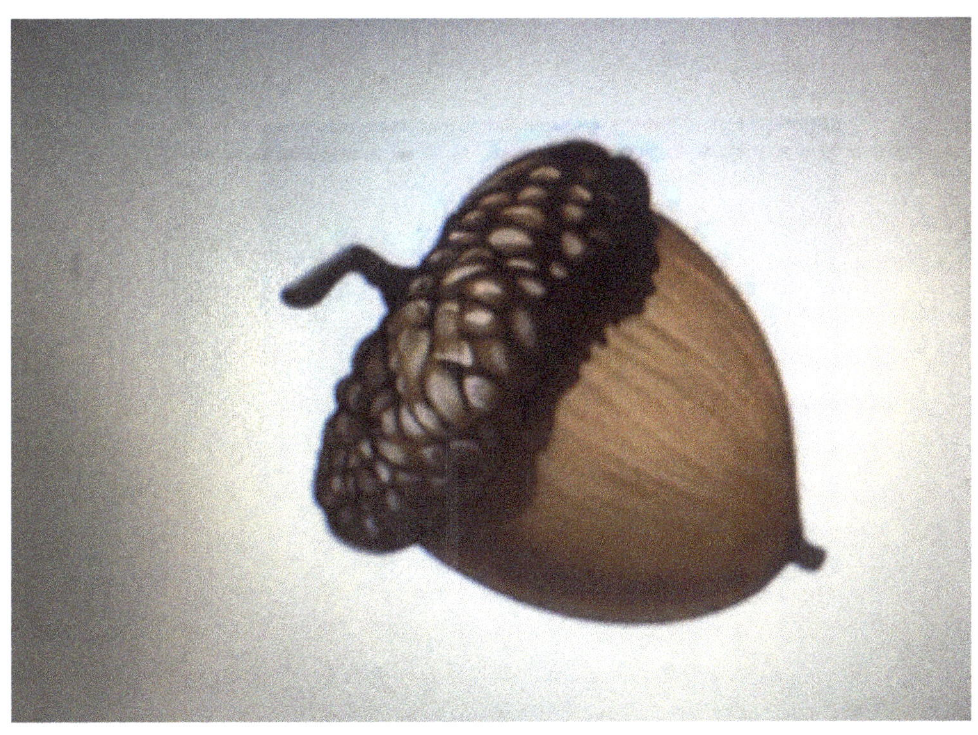

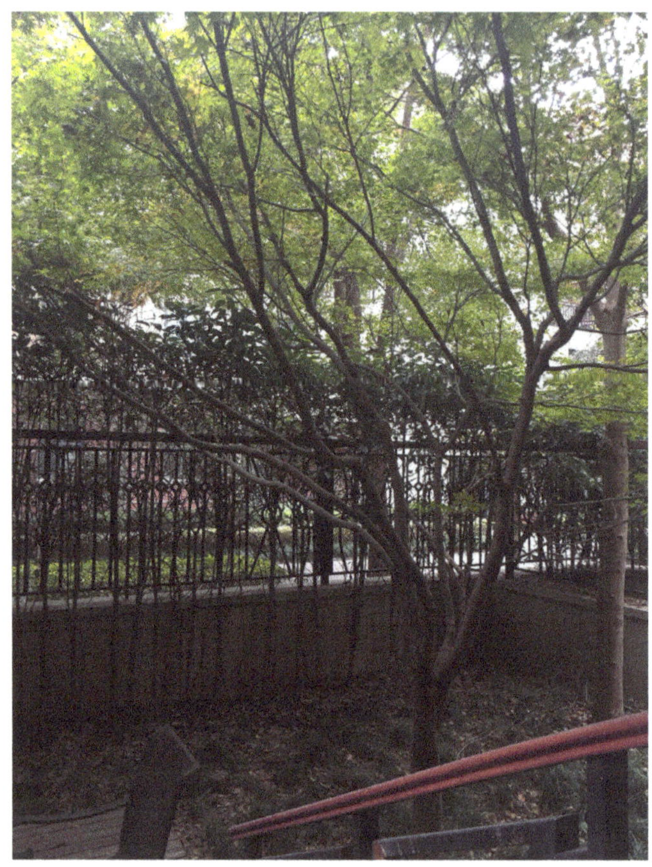

First off, I got to tell you I'm happy writing about this guy. Talk about growth. He is the acorn that becomes the oak tree. I instantly liked him from the moment I first met him. We didn't get close until some years later, which is great, because I got to know him so well. Almost twenty years now. The guy has always been there for me, as I have been for him. A solid and funny guy. He was known as Sprout. I thought he was more like a mushroom, because he's a fungi. Get It? Fun guy! Wheow.

It is time to tell you about Wheow. It's how he talks. Grunts actually. It's a universal word, because it works for anything. Yes, anything. It is the noise you make when getting out of bed in the morning. We all do it, but he turned it into his own language. We all learned this language and use it daily. I love telling people the story of my friend, Jason. Married to a lovely girl named Teresa. They have two kids and are great parents. Like I said, talk about growing and going. So, wheow!

# A Freebee!

- any kind of booze
- any flavor
- any size
- any shape
- any where
- any time
- any place
- any thing
- any temperature

We all have friends or relatives who are cheap, frugal, or thrifty. John is the original, where it all began. The expert. He has plenty of dough. He works hard and gets paid well, so there's no need for him to be that way. I think he simply gets a kick out of it, as I do. It sure isn't boring being around him.

Sometimes we love it when we get a deal or a good price; however, it makes his year—not day—even though he does it on a daily basis. I could tell you many stories, but there are too many.

Now that I said how cheap he is, it's time to let you behind the curtain. He would do just about anything for me. You've heard the term, "he would give you the shirt off his back"? That's him, and he would probably just buy you a new one. The man is golden when it comes to helping people. I believe it's in his DNA to be helpful, and that is rare. I'm totally grateful to have him as a friend. One last thing, I know he'd stop on a dime to help anyone or to pick up that dime!

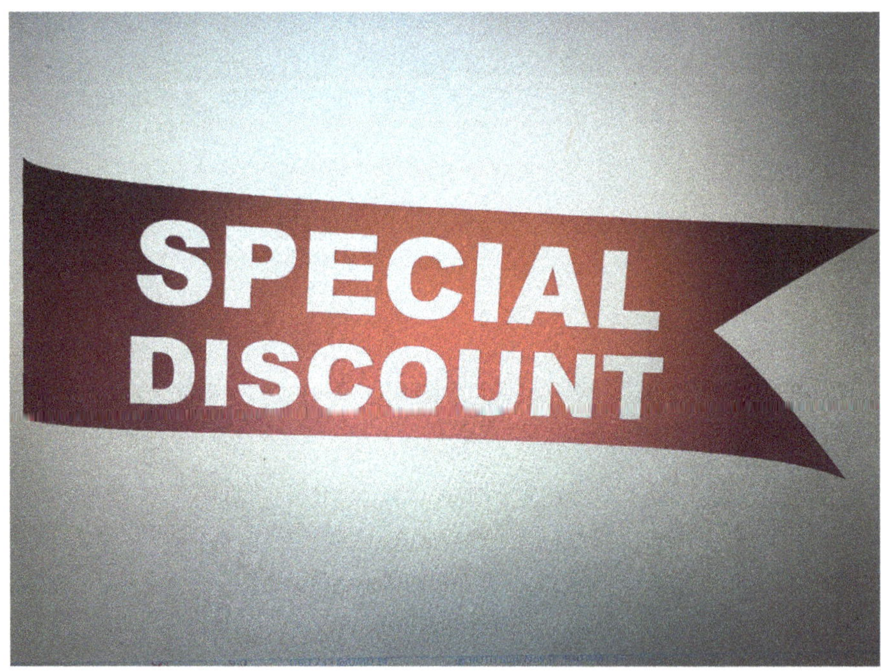

# Keir Erin

- ► 4 oz Crown Royal whiskey
- ► 2 oz Merlyn Cream Liqueur
- ► rocks glass with ice

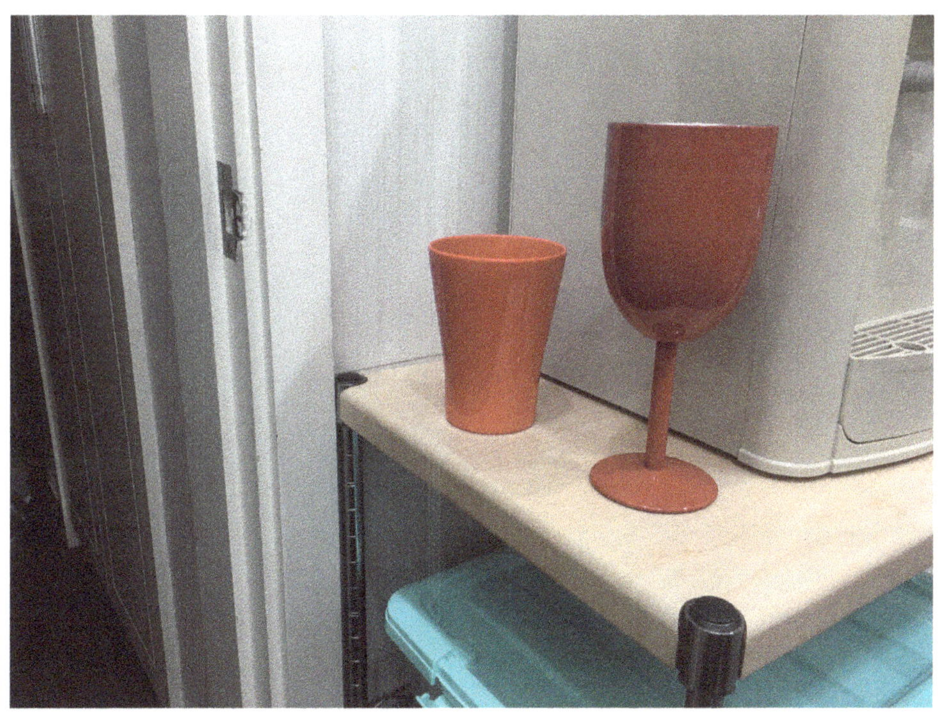

We all have friends who are couples. Some are my wife's my co-workers and their spouses, and some are mine. However, it's not always a perfect match, nor should it be. But this one couple is close enough to perfect for us. Truth be told, we really don't hang out with them often. It's okay, we really just need great couples friends in this world. Oh, I'm talking about Erin and Keiron here. He's from Wales (not the mammal), and she's from Canada. I don't know why that matters, but I find it interesting because I'm from a different planet, and my wife is from earth. Okay, back to the story.

All of us lived in Qatar at the same time but didn't know each other, which I find strange because it's such a small country. I'd like to believe that our paths did cross at some point, like at a bar or the rugby club. I can imagine our conversation now. The guys are talking sports. The girls talking shop. All of us getting along so well. Now we live in China in the same building. Coincidence?

# Junior Drink

Vodka mixed with a fruity, sweet, or girlie liquid. Yes, really: girlie!

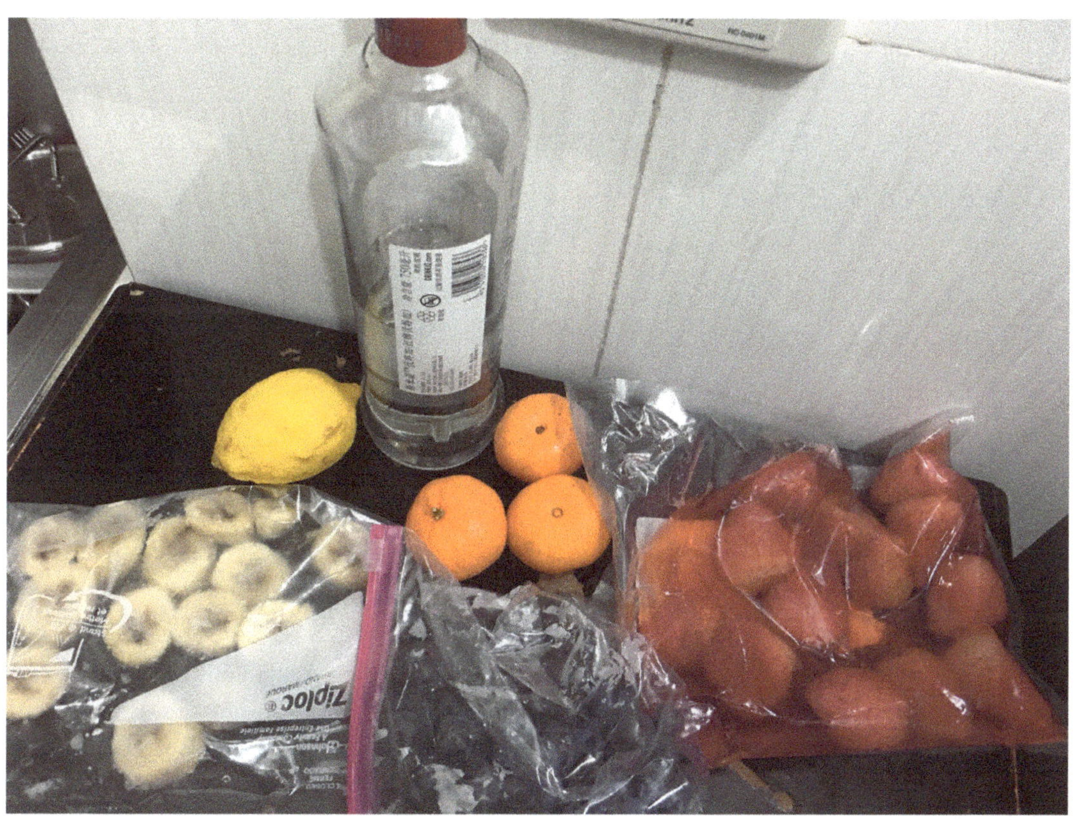

Okay, this is my junior, Jeremy. I'm already getting weepy now. Not just because he's my junior, but also because I have way too many fond and monumental memories. Classic! Friends for twenty years. I could write a whole book on our adventures, but I'll start with why I call him Junior.

When I met this young man, believe it or not, he was really shy. He was a server, and I was a bartender at the same restaurant. I was asked who we should make bartender next. I suggested Jeremy, to which the boss laughed at me. "He's too quiet," he said. I said, "No, you wait for him to come out of his shell, and then look out, for he's got a little something there." Well, I got my way as I often do, but I was wrong.

He was awful, really awful. He was only good at filling the ice bin. Hence, "ice junior" was the phrase used to get him to move or be motivated. Now over time, Junior became quite the worker, bartender, and man! I mentioned twenty years of friendship with him. It's actually twenty years of family!

# A Big Al

- 4 oz rum
- 2 oz triple sec
- 2 oz blue curaçao
- splash of sour mix
- splash of pineapple
- wedge of lemon
- pint glass filled with ice

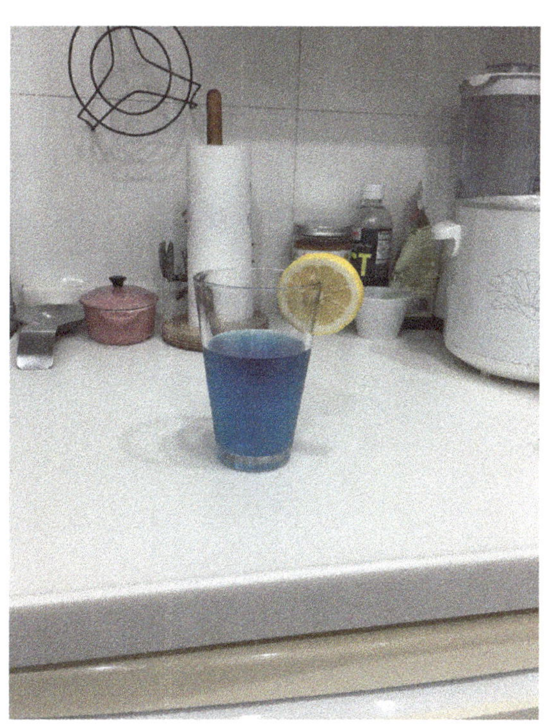

This drink is blue in color. Al is never blue in life, bra!

I often thought of myself as a pretty good guy. Funny and generous. Two qualities I admire in people. I'm saddened and ecstatic that my friend, Al, makes me look silly when it comes to being a viable person in this world. As I've said many times before, it is needed. He fills this position by being himself. I can't see any flaws in him. His wife, Gin Slim, might disagree. Ha! We met in China and instantly became lifelong friends. His wife and daughters, Shawna and Emma, too. My wife approves. Why do I need her stamp of approval? I am smart, that's why!

I have *one* story I want to tell, for it best describes this man. At school, when asked about a class that is not offered to students, his response was that if someone is willing to apply themselves to better themselves, then we should offer it. Wow! A good guy does that for humanity. No, a *great* guy! An example setter for living. Most people don't live that way, so keep being you, all right?

# A Canadian Cocktail

- 4 oz Canadian whiskey
- 2 oz triple sec
- 2 oz soda water
- splash of sour mix
- wedge of lemon
- pint glass

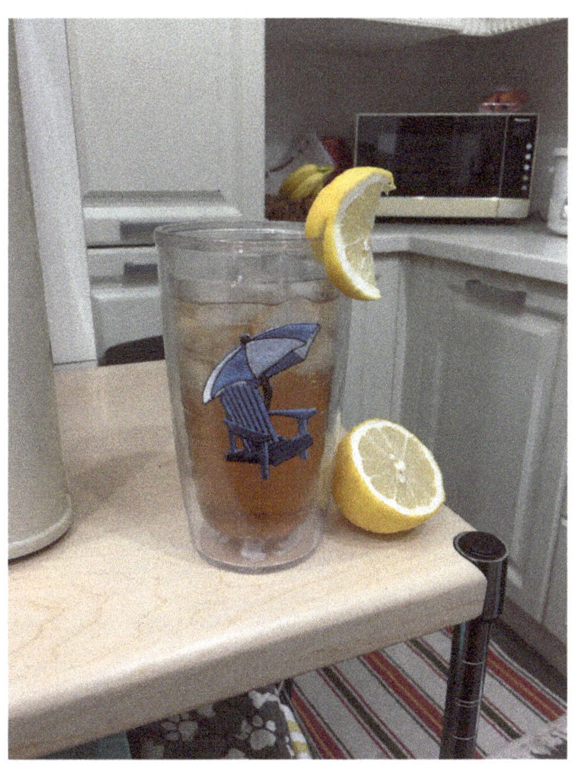

You know, perception is a big deal in our life these days. More often than not, we are wrong about people, but I'm not mistaken about my buddy, Scott. A finer man you will never meet. They say his job defines him. It's quite a demanding job requiring integrity, decency, patience, and, of course, knowledge. I say Scott defines the job, not the other way around. The opposite. Also, people say he is a pushover. Well, again, he is not. He simply knows how to handle things. He and I often have one-on-one conversations about many things, and he says they help him out.

Truth be told, it helps *me* out more. I quote this phrase: "He makes me want to be a better man." Again, the opposite. I'm not liking the term opposite. It's more so, an awesome dude. A great gift to mankind. One more example. His wife, Amy, and son, Blake, are both awesome as well. He says they make him a better man. I believe it goes both ways. Right as rain, bra!

# A-V

Jameson and Ginger

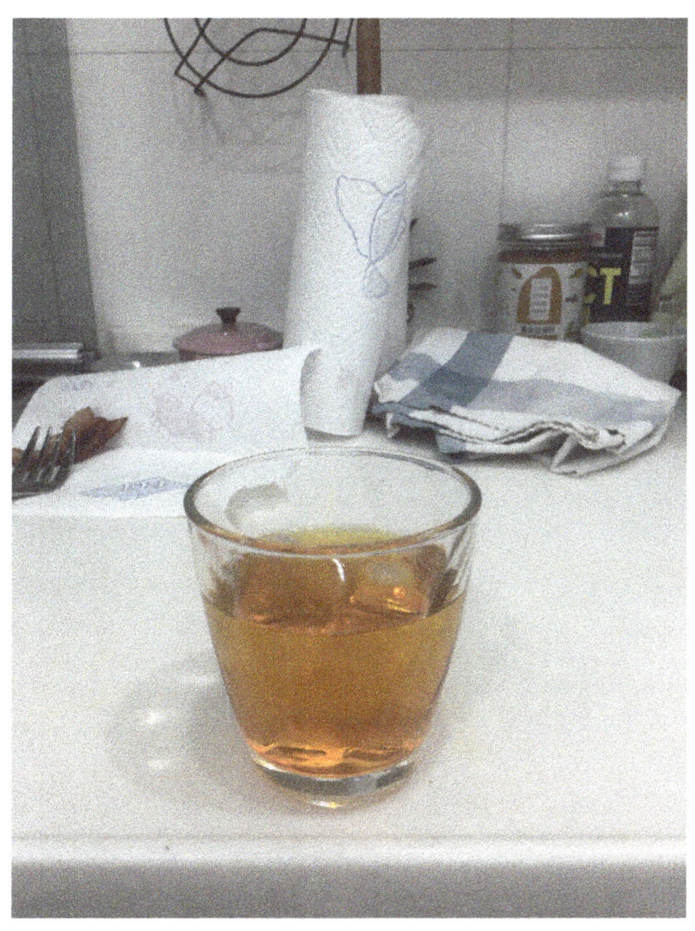

Mikey V. My main man, Mikey V. My friend and my *la famiglia*. My bra. I played the most golf with this guy. My favorite thing. On the golf course is where you get to know people the best. His impressions of Crazy Pants Johnson and his straw hat are two fine examples. Also, his impression of me is spot on as his award-winning personality. I've known him going on twenty years now. A calm, patient man with an awful lot of wit and humor. He also reinvents himself often while staying the same charming self. Again, my bra.

He and I worked together off and on for many years. He married the love of his life on a bad weather day, which didn't seem to faze him at all. A go-with-the-flow kind of guy. To this day he adores Kim, his bride, I know for sure! How do I know? Because he told me, and he lives it. Now why Jameson and Ginger? Well Kim and V could both change their names to Jameson and Ginger and become those people. They are that much fun. Love you two!

# Review Requested:

If you loved this book, would you please provide
a review at Amazon.com?